DEDICATION

This book is dedicated to all of my former students who have become pediatric practitioners. The most any teacher can hope for is to inspire others to make the world a better place- and you do, EVERY DAY. Thank you Healthcare Heroes!

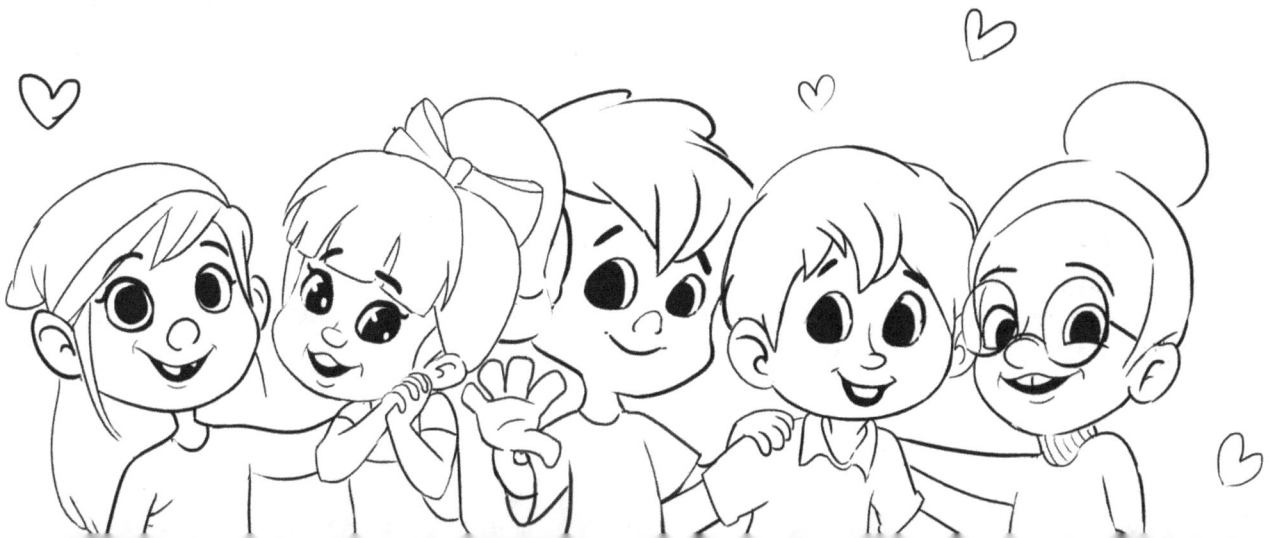

PREFACE

Who ever heard of a preface in a children's book? I am a healthcare educator and I want to share a couple of thoughts with you parents, grandparents, nannies, and big siblings before you read this book with your little one.

First, in spite of the title, this is not a book to invalidate children's real and justified anxieties about a new experience. When kids are nervous, parents often say, "It will be fine! There's nothing to be afraid of." My suggestion is not to shut the child down, but validate those feelings and offer a model way of dealing with them. Dad could say, "I know, bud, I was nervous last time I went to the doctor but that's how we stay healthy."

Second, never under-estimate the power of magical thinking. Remember when you could fly? Take those fun, whimsical analogies and apply them to situations that are causing anxiety. My favorite one in here is the "Super Power Detector." As a paramedic on the ambulance, I was usually assured of a super power score over 90. WHAT A POWERFUL KID!

Third, never lie to children about what you suspect might be part of the visit. Especially when there is a chance of that dreaded SHOT! Being straightforward will help build trust, and ensure that your child won't feel betrayed or blindsided if things don't go as planned.

Next, manage your own anxiety. After over 30 years in healthcare, I have found that the child's reaction is directly proportional to the caretaker's. You can be your pediatrician's best asset or worst nightmare. If your little one isn't having any of that Ear Light, volunteer to have it demonstrated on you. Your steady example is golden.

And last, if your child is having difficulty expressing worries, try helping narrow down the source of "I'm scared." What are they uncomfortable with? If it is the unknown, have some empathy. We're all afraid of the unknown. Try a conversation like, "Let's talk about what's going to happen tomorrow, step by step. Say stop when we get to something that sounds scary.. We can talk about how to make it less scary before we go."....And read this book! Hope it helps.

Sometimes you get sick

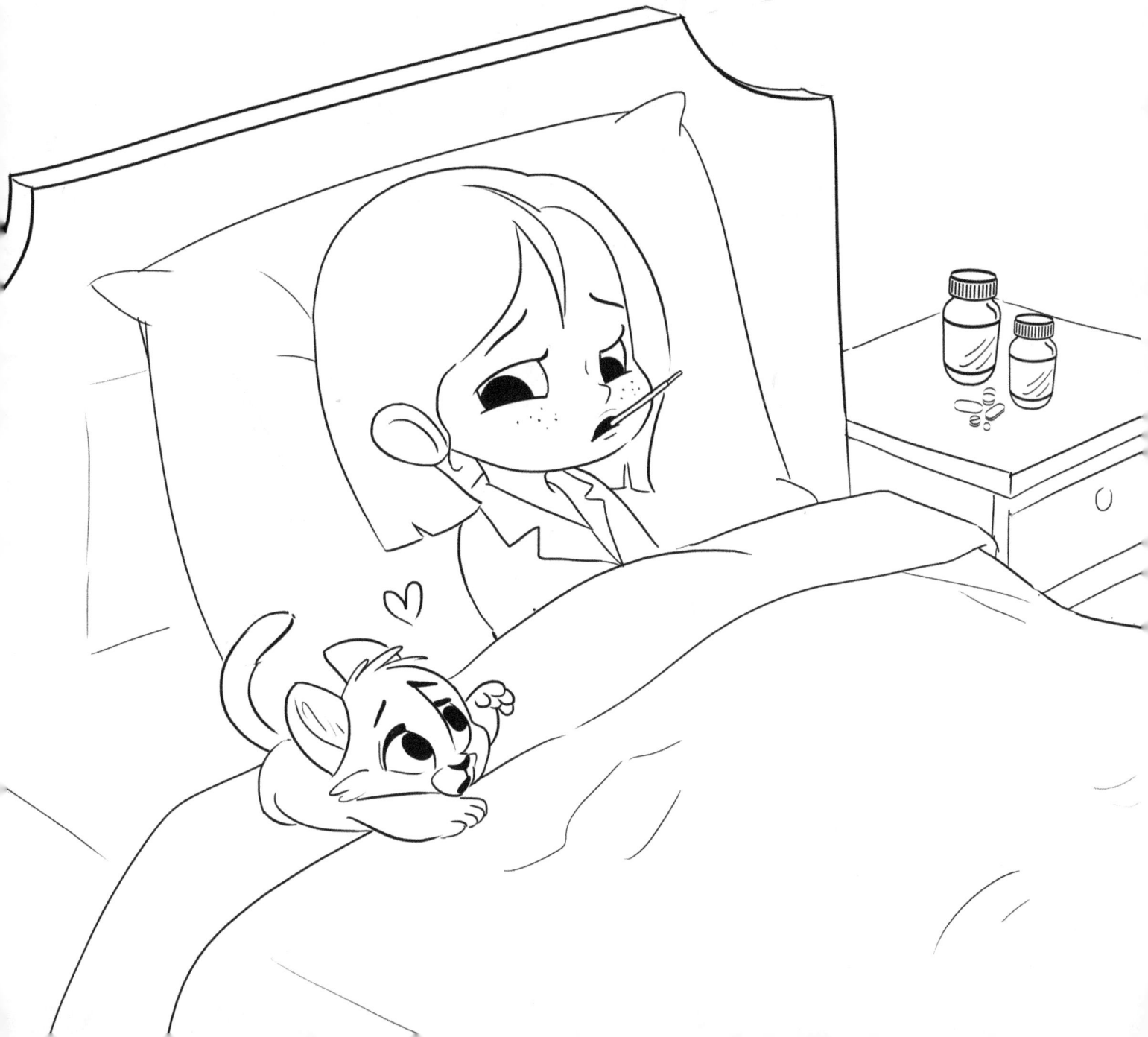

You could get a scratch
or scrape,

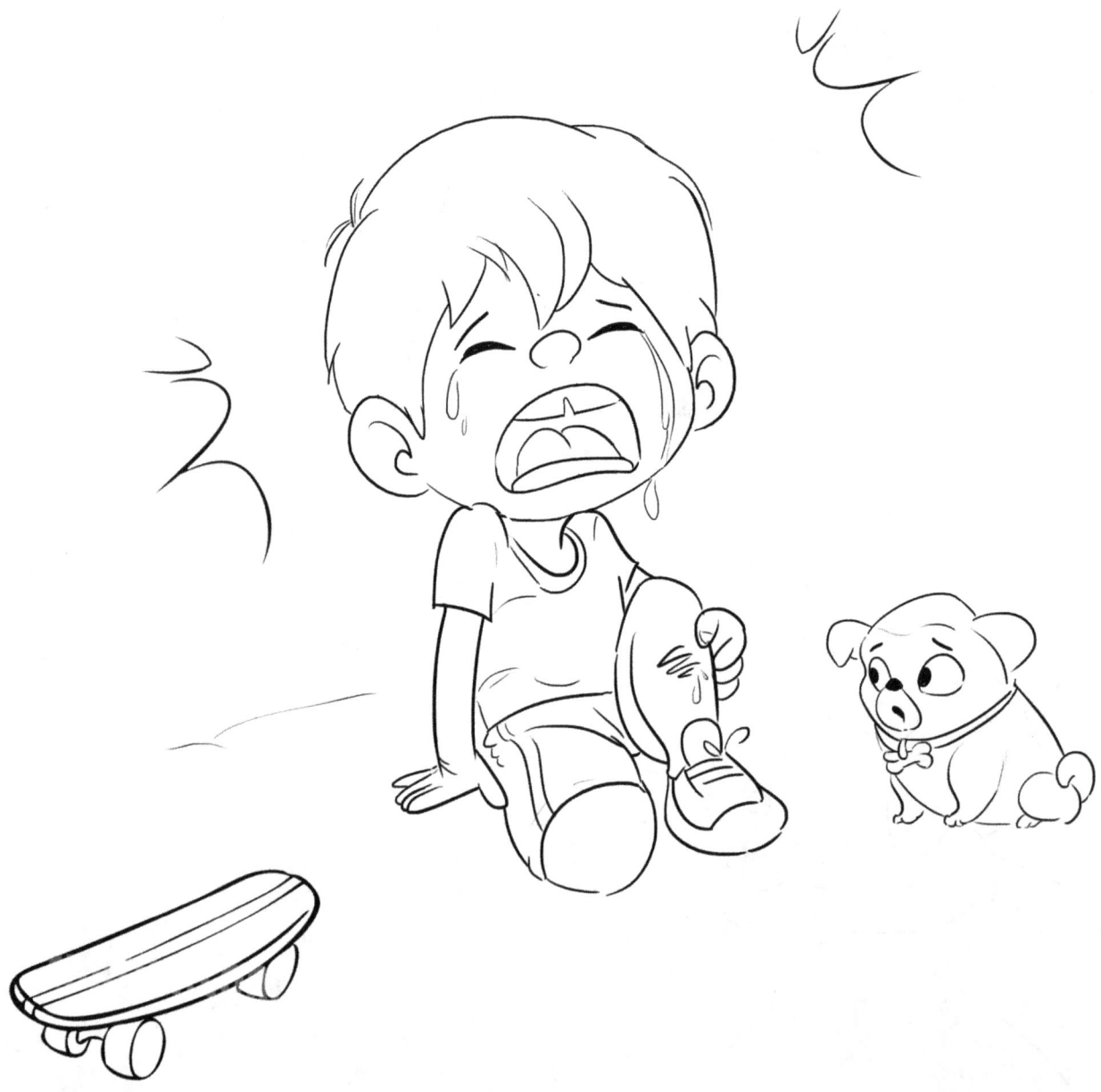

or even break a bone!

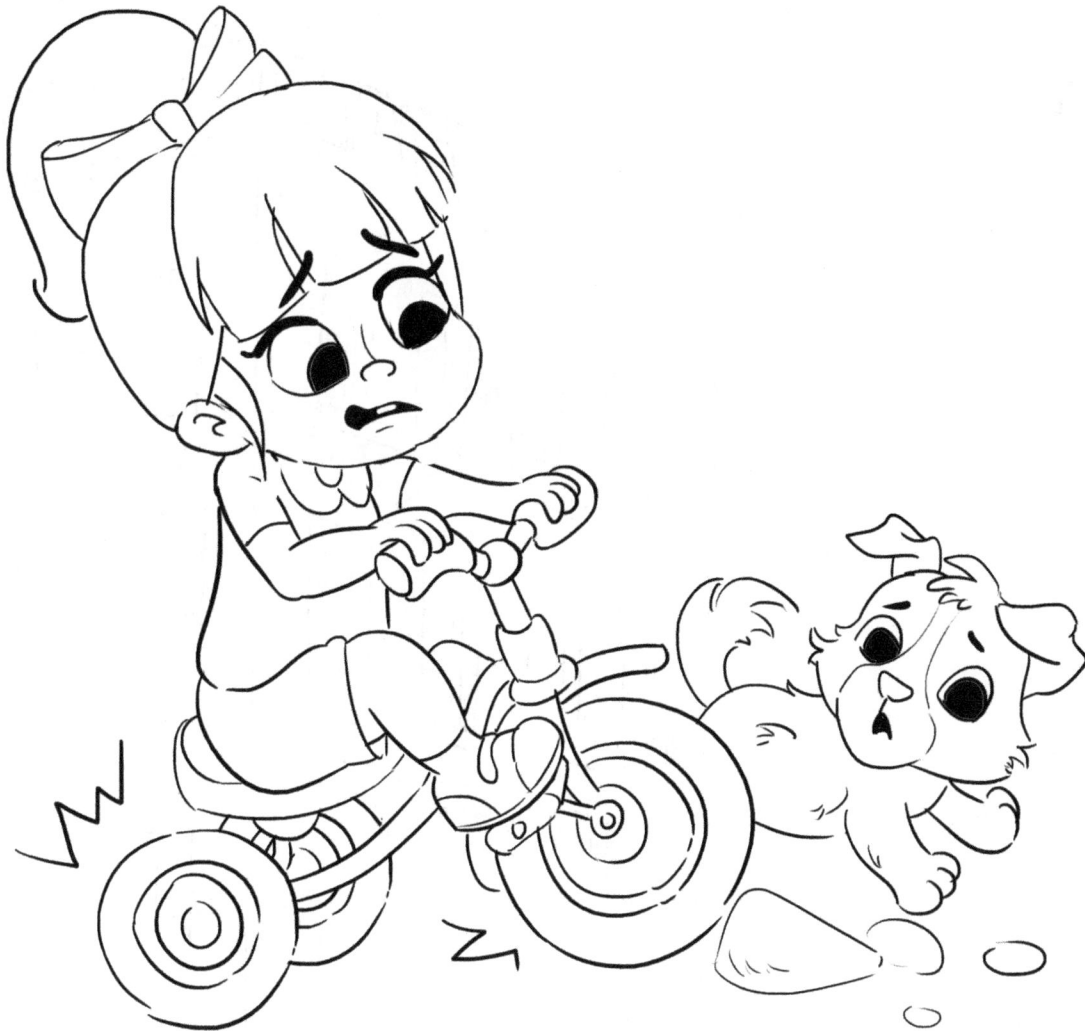

When this happens, you might take
a trip to a doctor or a hospital.

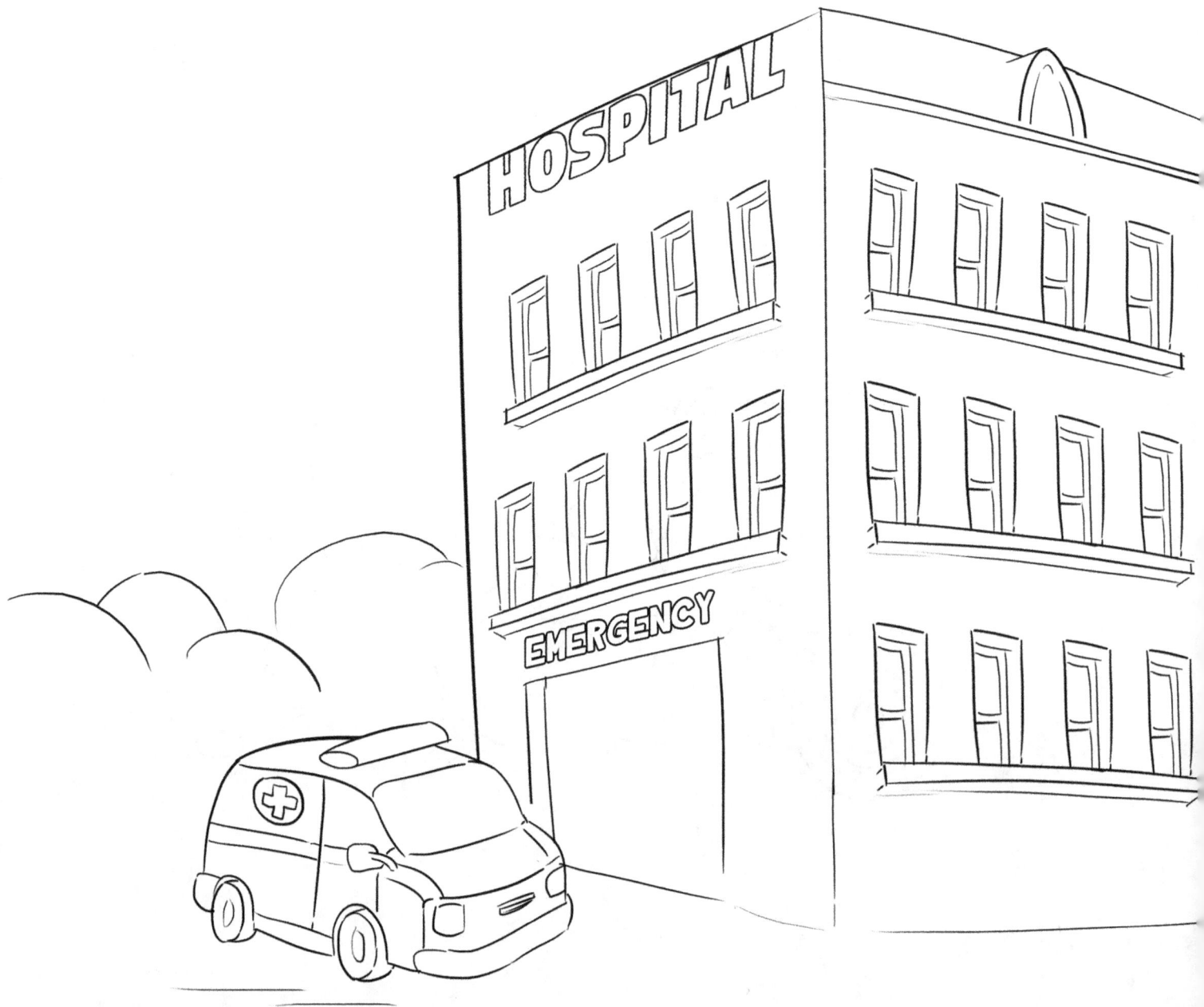

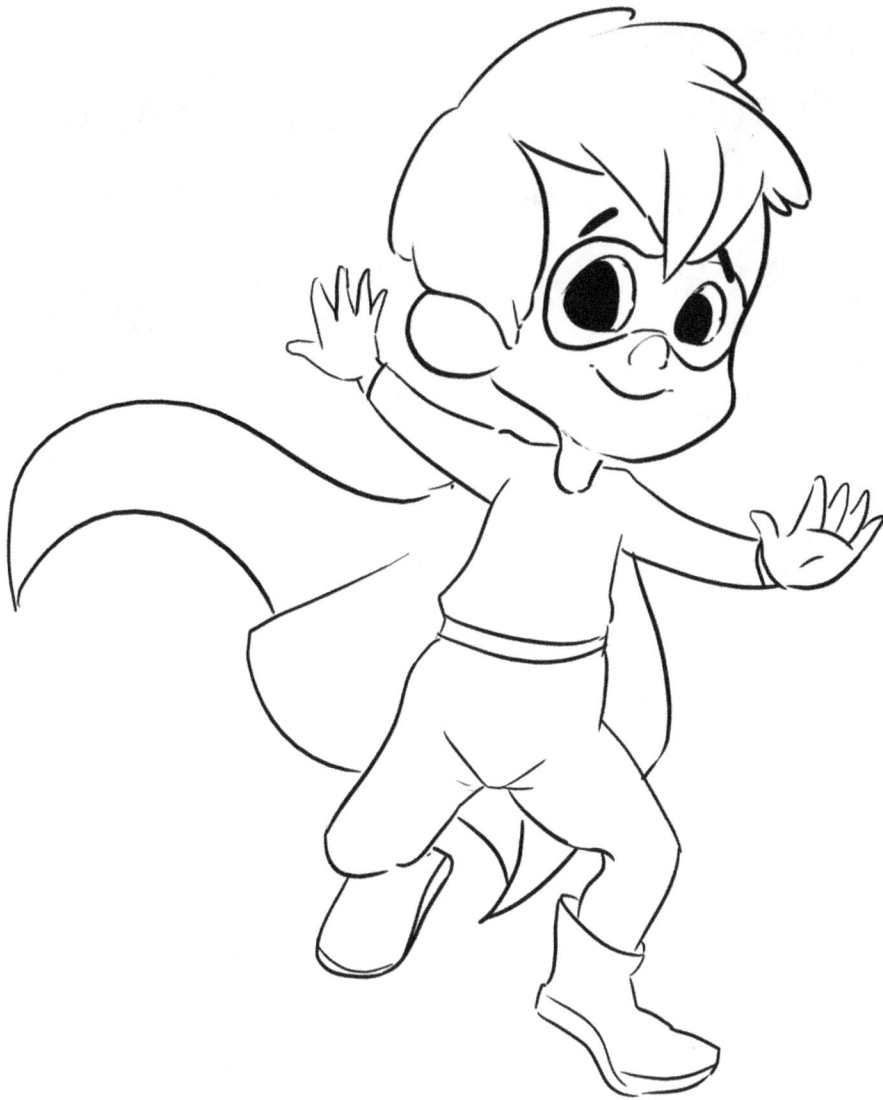

This book tells you what happens
there so it won't be SCARY.
Even your mom or dad could be nervous,
so read this book with them and help them be brave.

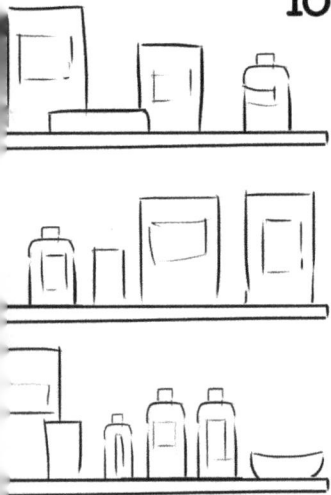

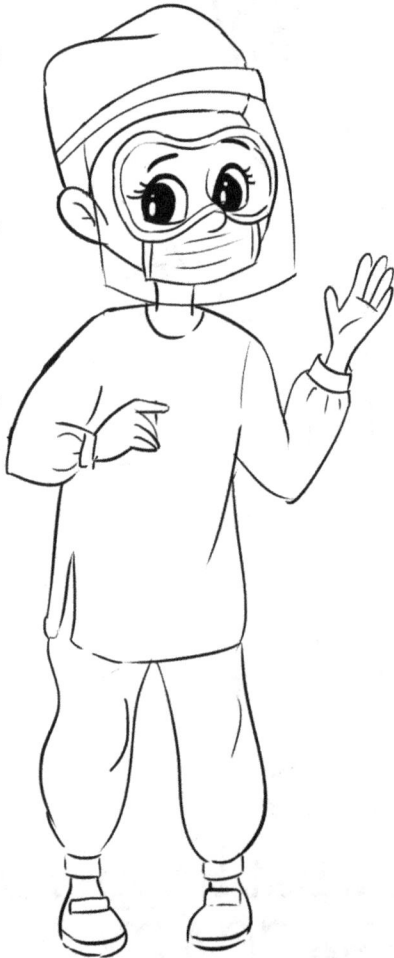

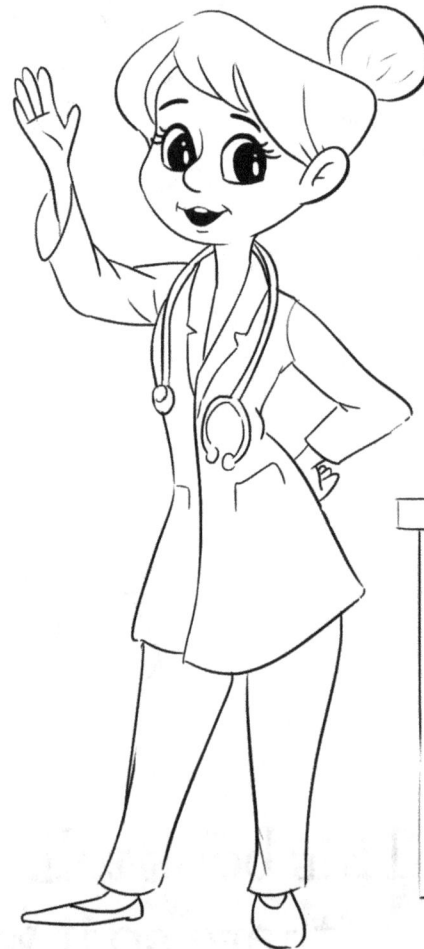

THE ROBOT SCALE

Stand on the funny robot scale
to see if you're getting bigger!

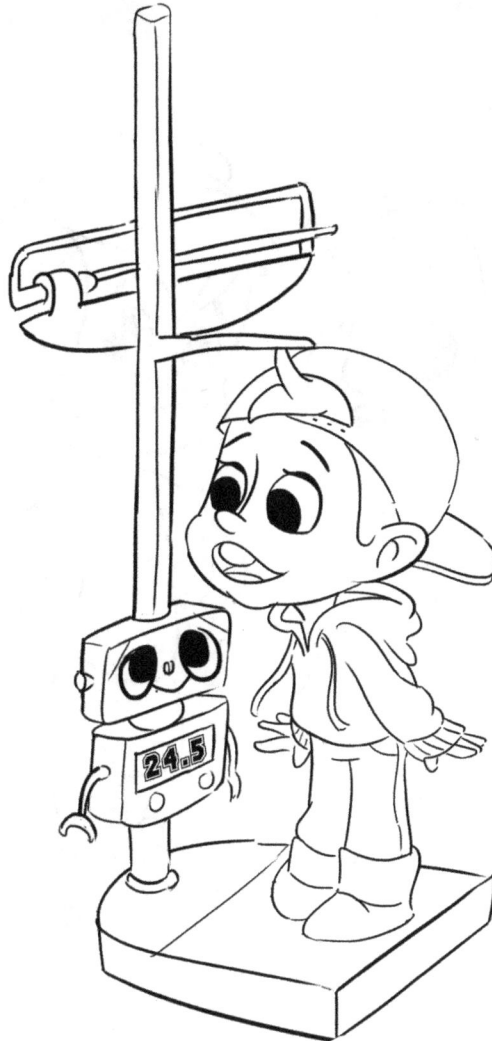

24.5

NOT SCARY!

X-RAYS

PICTURE TIME! This is you on the outside

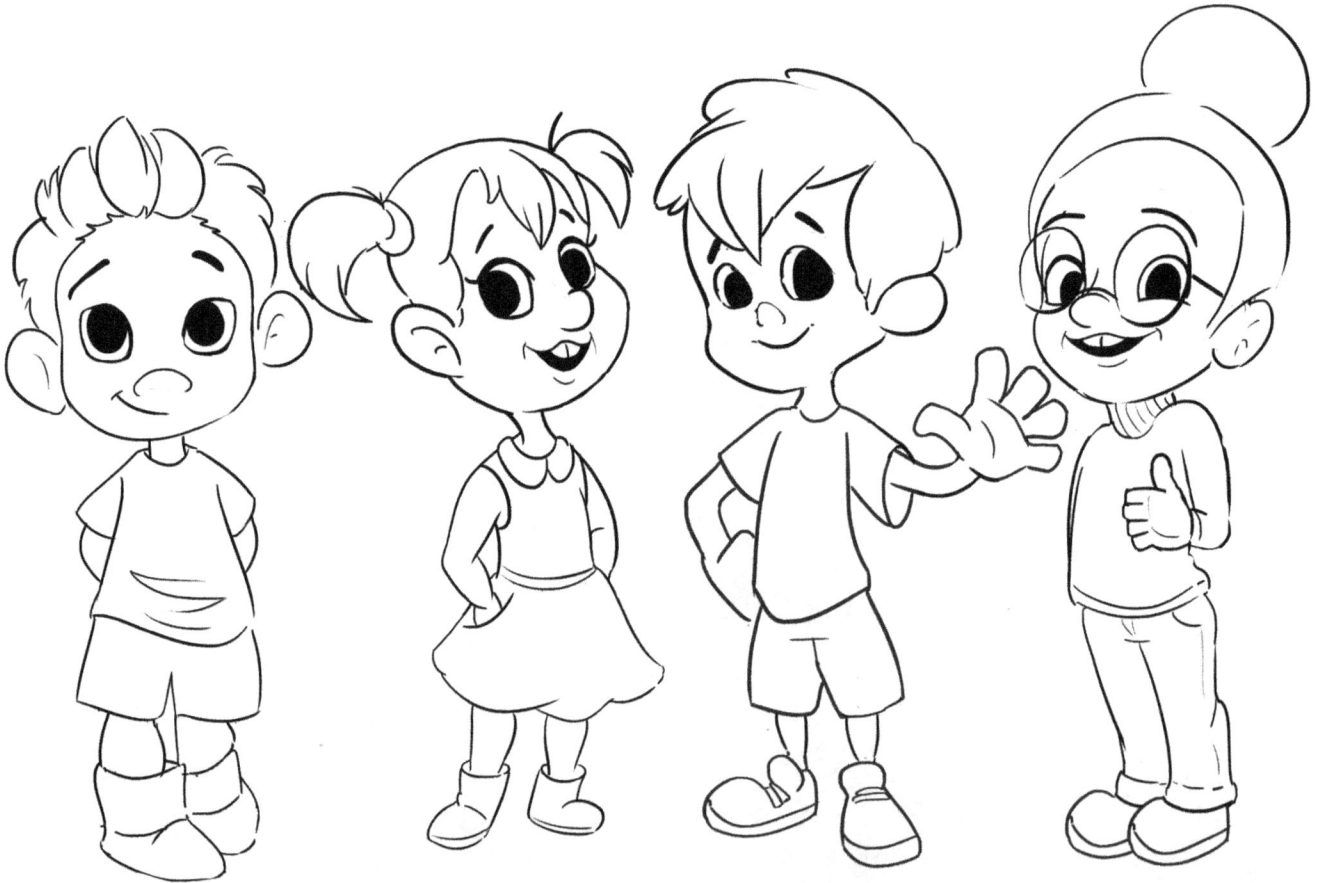

This is you on the inside. We can't see you on the inside without a special machine. It's called an X-RAY.
It doesn't hurt a bit, but you have to hold really still so they can take a good picture.

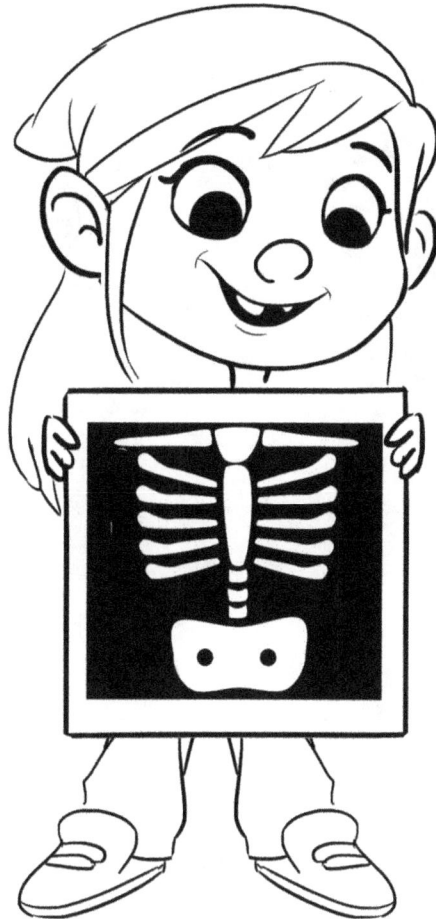

NOT SCARY!
Say cheese!

SHOTS

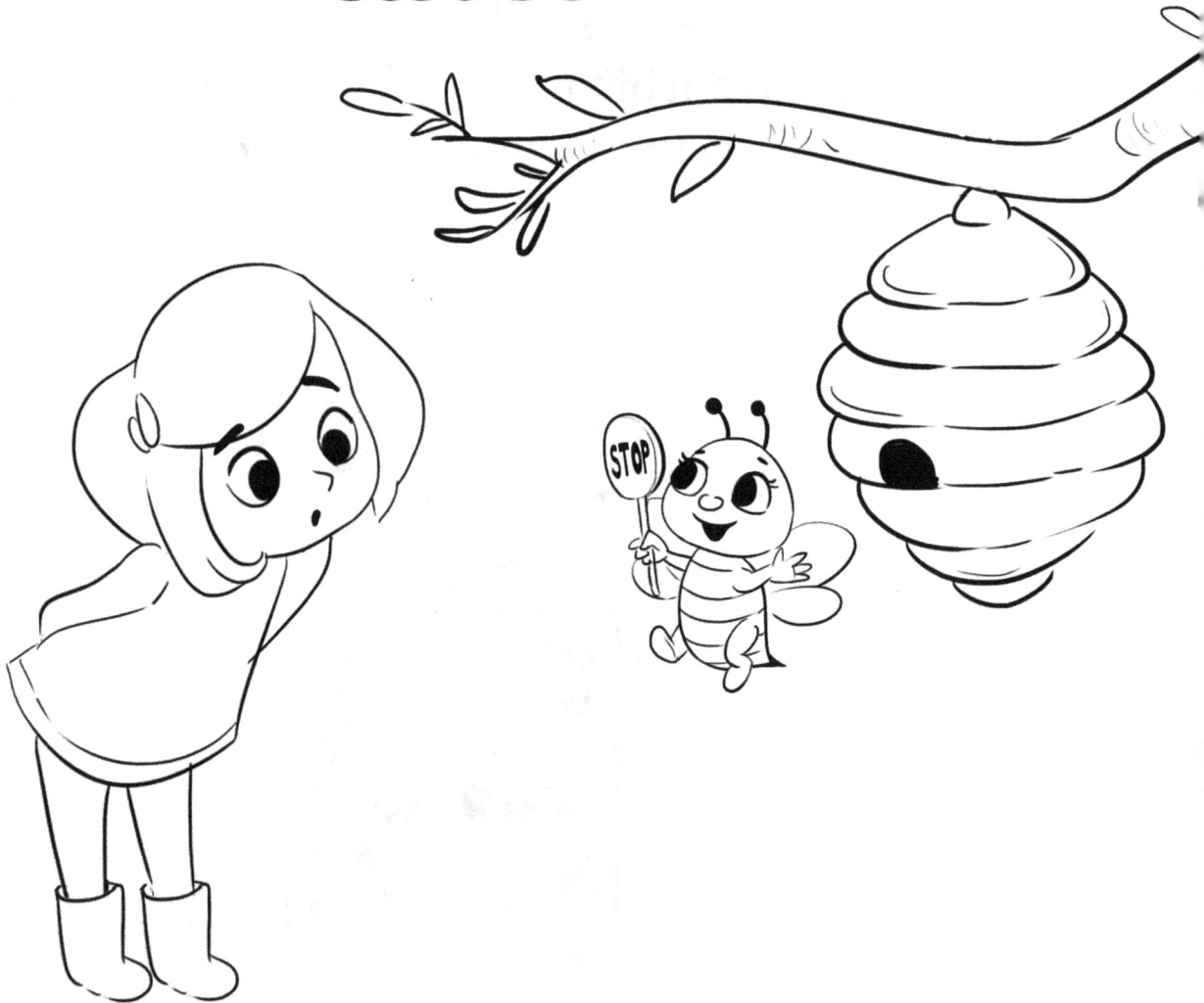

When a bee wants you to leave her home or food alone,
she might stick you with her stinger to make you go away.
"OUCH! That hurts!"
...but not too bad, and not for very long. You can be brave.

Sometimes you need some medicine to make you better, or to keep you from getting sick. That medicine has to go under your skin so they use a thing with a point called a needle. You can tell your parents the nurse gave you a

SHOT

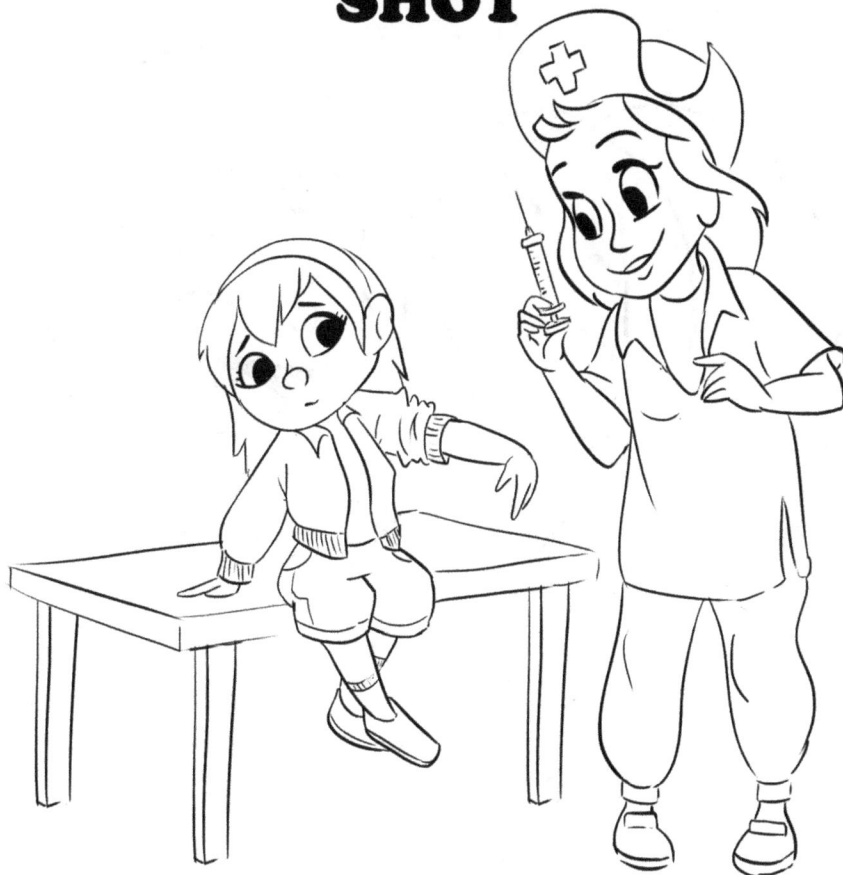

"OUCH! That hurts!"...but not too bad, and not for long.

A LITTLE SCARY BUT...

You can be brave.

THE ARM HUGGER
(blood pressure cuff)

Everyone loves a big, warm hug.

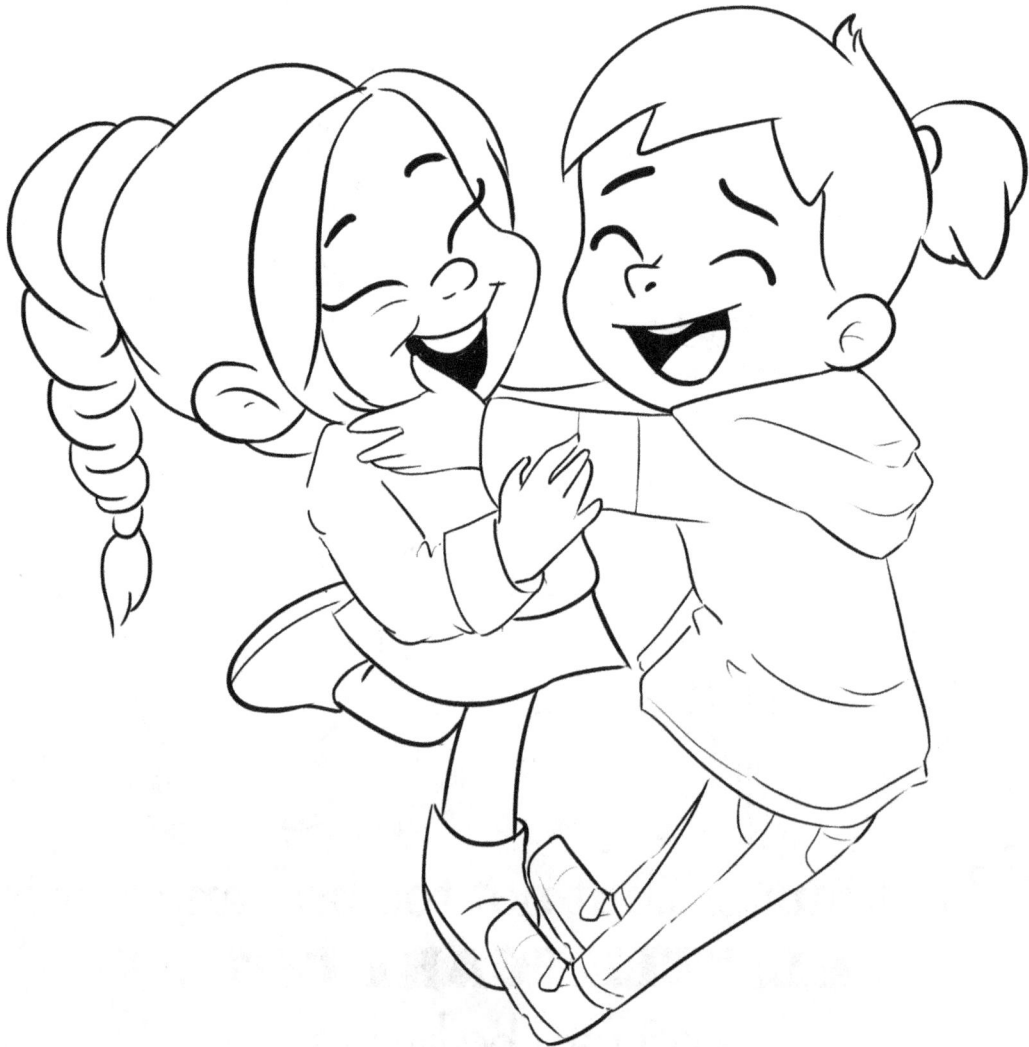

At your doctor's office, sometimes they use this silly-looking "blood pressure cuff" to give your arm a hug. Like this

NOT SCARY!

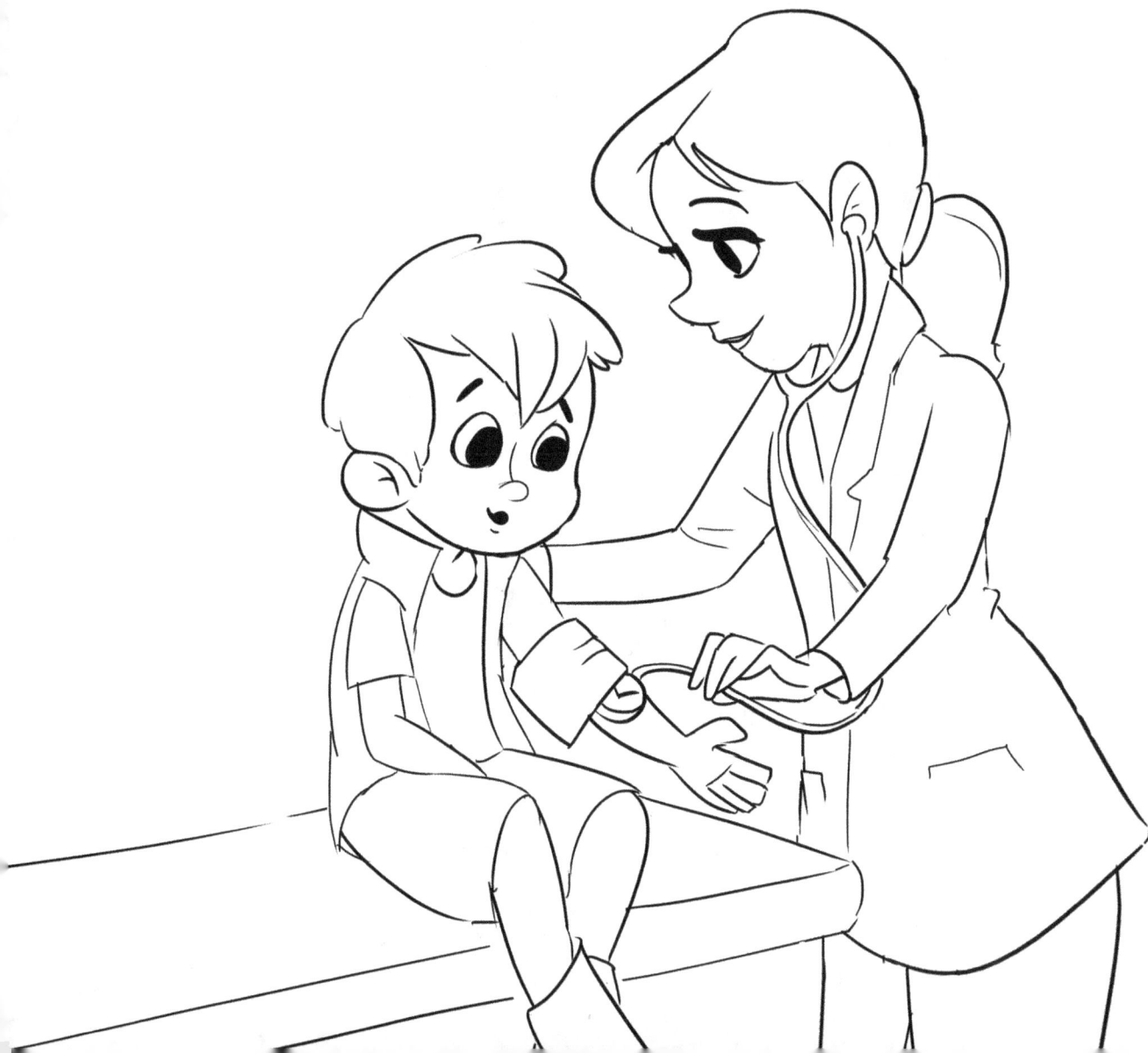

THE EAR LIGHT
(otoscope)

Have you ever played with a flashlight?

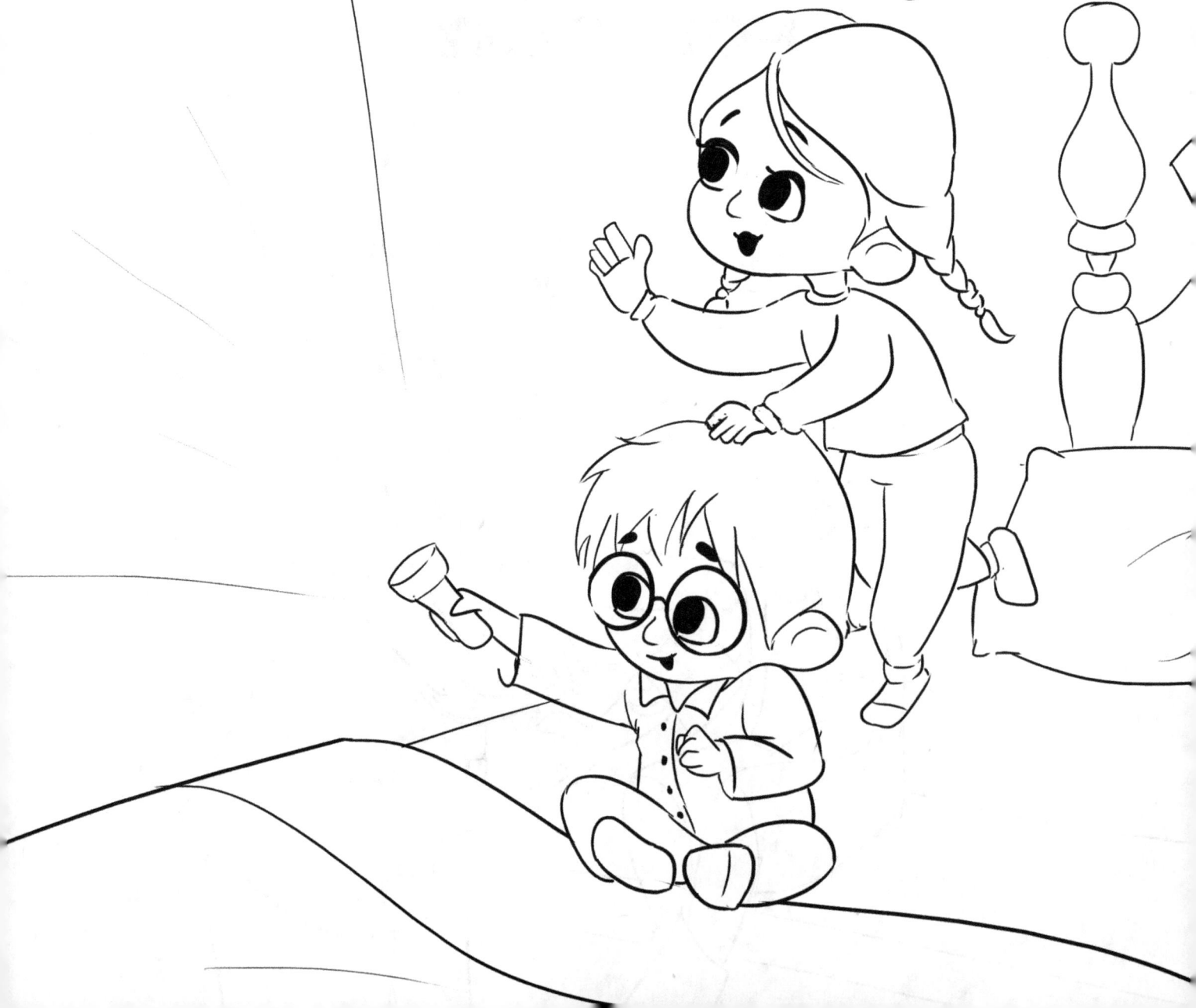

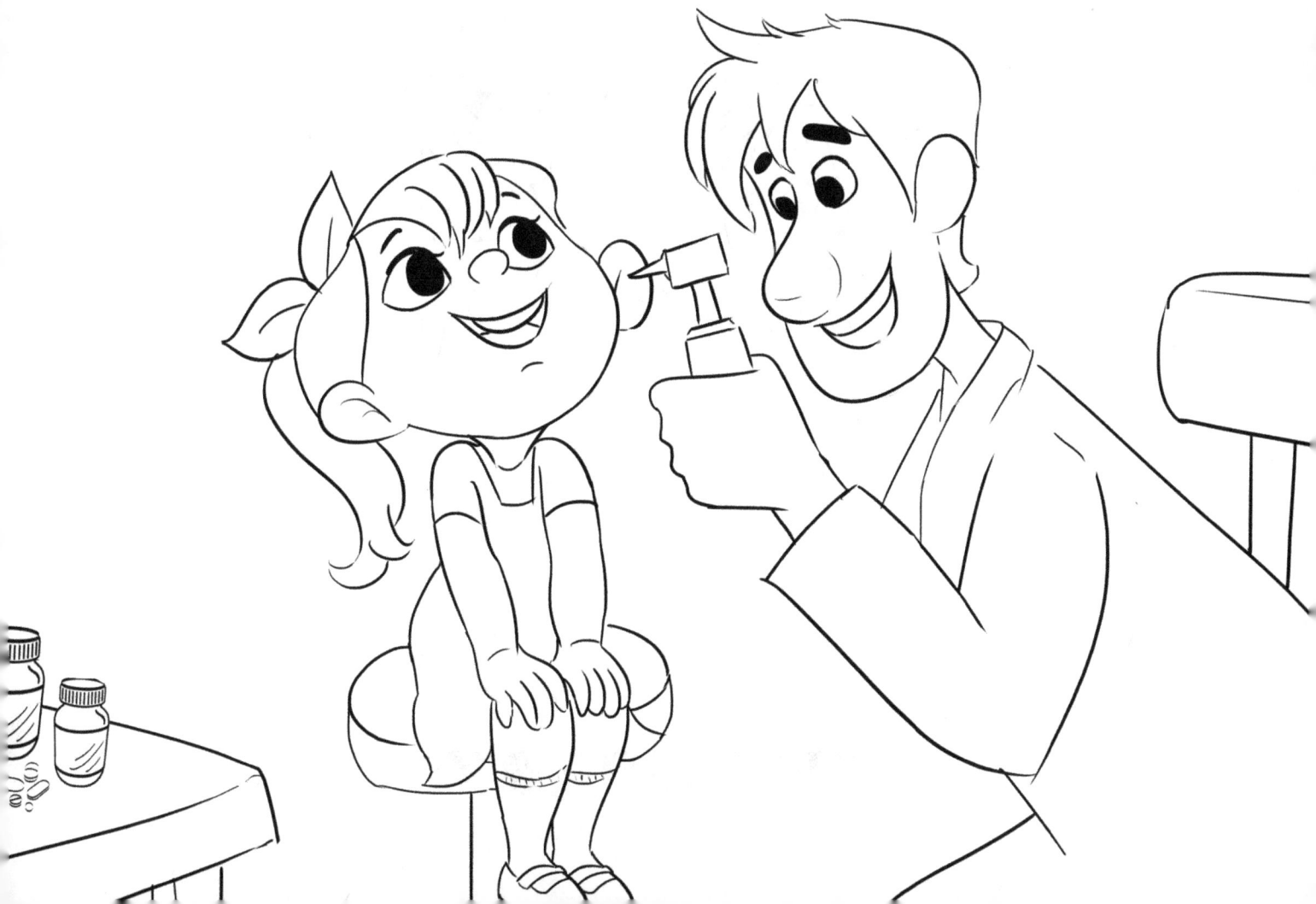

It's dark inside of your ears and nose
so the doctor uses a special flashlight to see what's in there!
(But don't YOU put anything in your ears or nose!)

NOT SCARY!

THE SUPER POWER DETECTOR
(pulse oximeter)

This is a super power detector. You put your finger inside and it tells you how strong your powers are... try to get a big number by taking a big deep breath. What's your score?

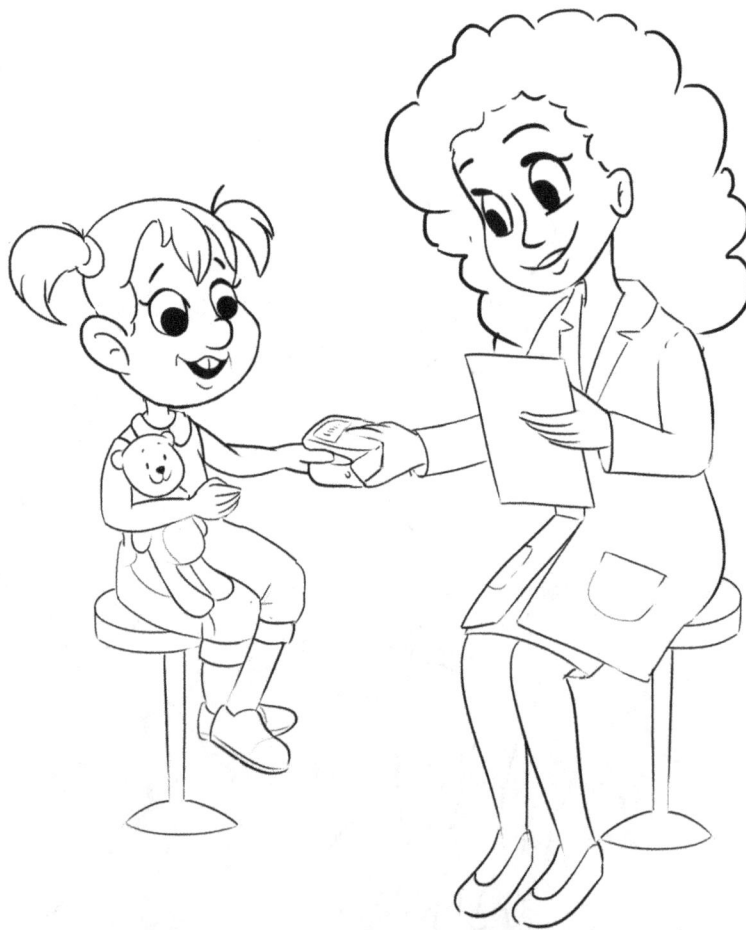

NOT SCARY!

DRAGON STEAM
(nebulizer/breathing treatment)

Do you like dragons?

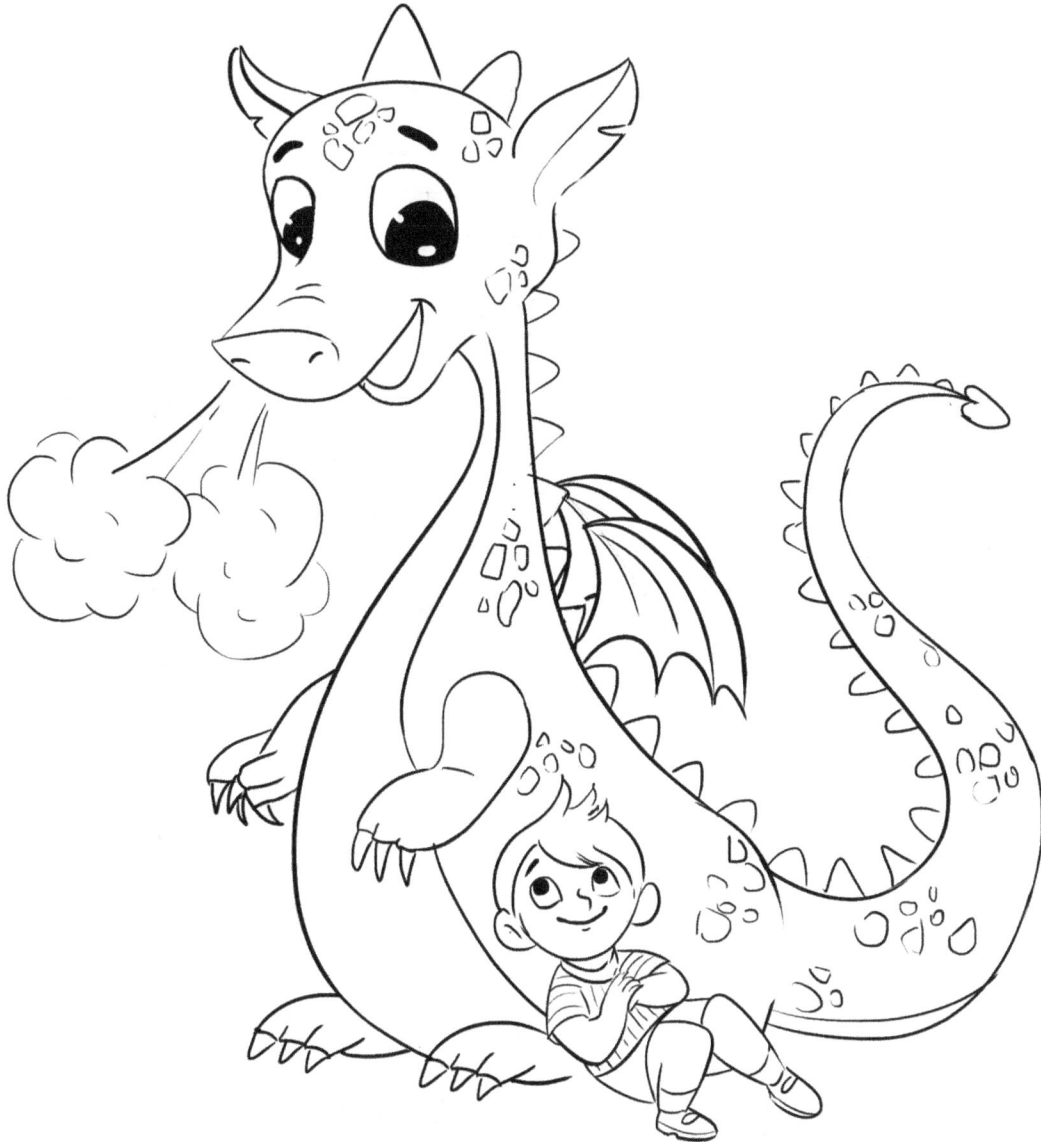

Sometimes you need a medicine that makes you breathe steam like a dragon. Take big deep breaths and make lots of clouds! Have fun and feel better!

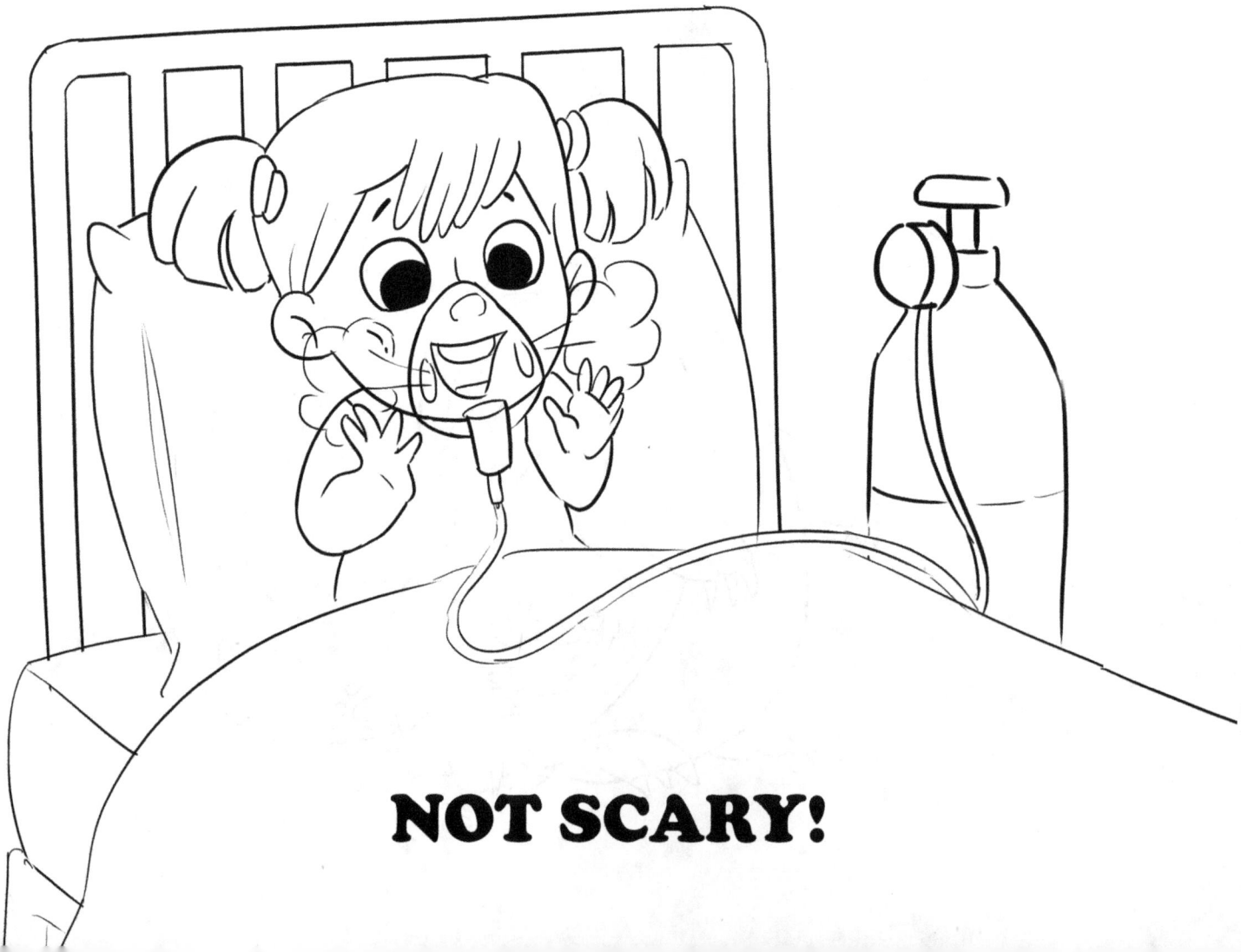

NOT SCARY!

STETHOSCOPE

Where is your heart?
Have you ever heard it beat?

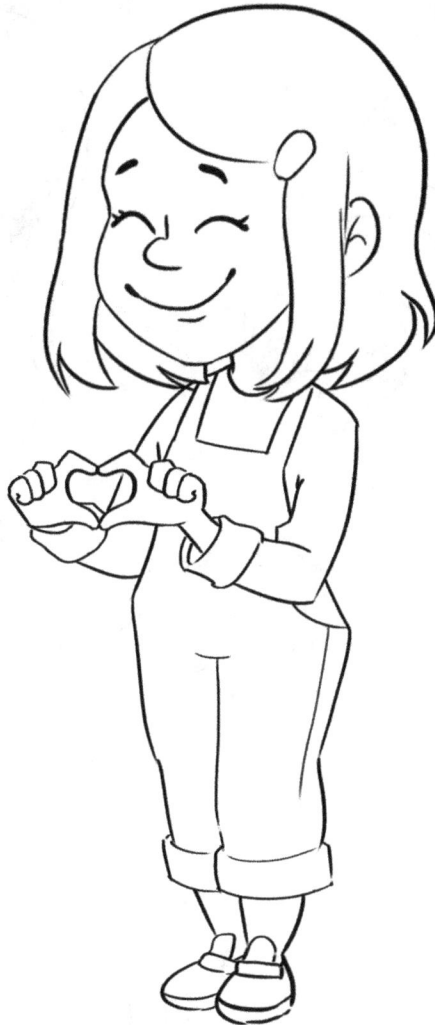

"Lub Dub, Lub Dub"

To hear your heart, you need one of these!

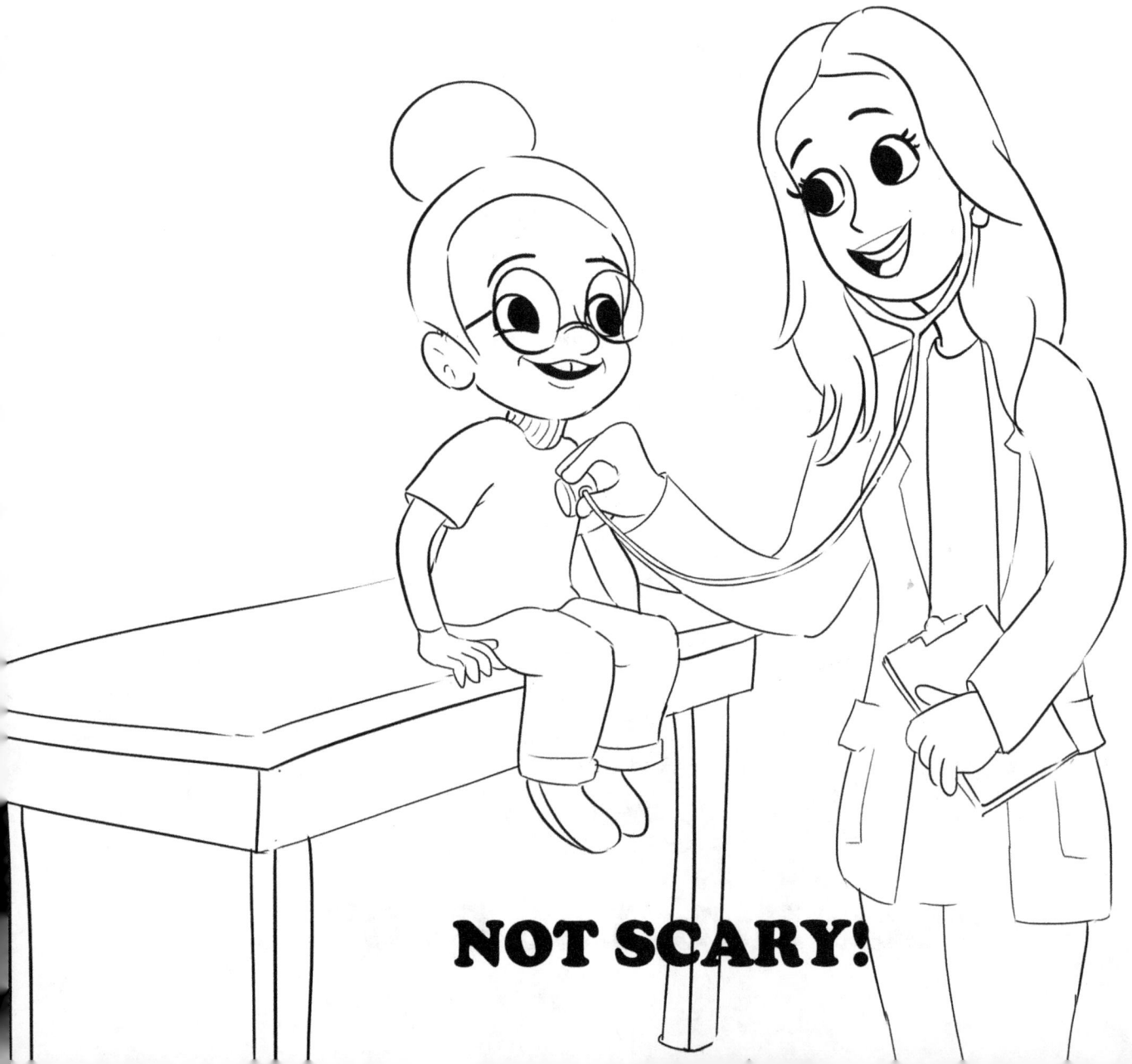

NOT SCARY!

MAGIC WAND
(reflex hammer)

Fairies, magicians, and wizards have magic wands to make surprising things happen.

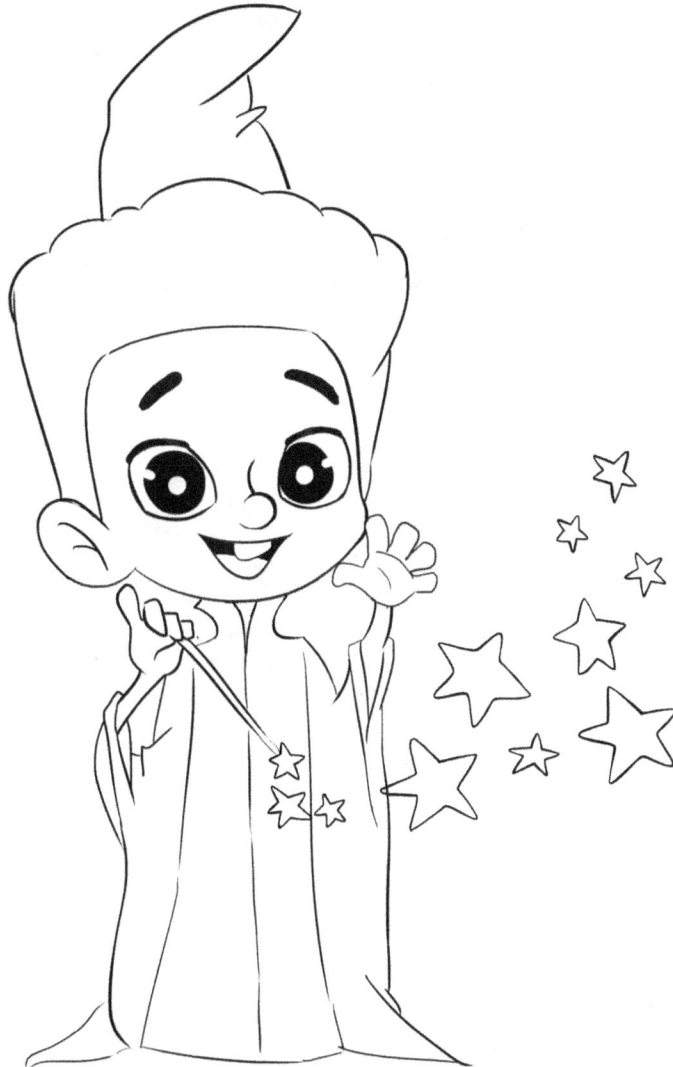

Your doctor has a wand that looks like this. One tap on your knee makes your leg move by itself! How funny to watch!

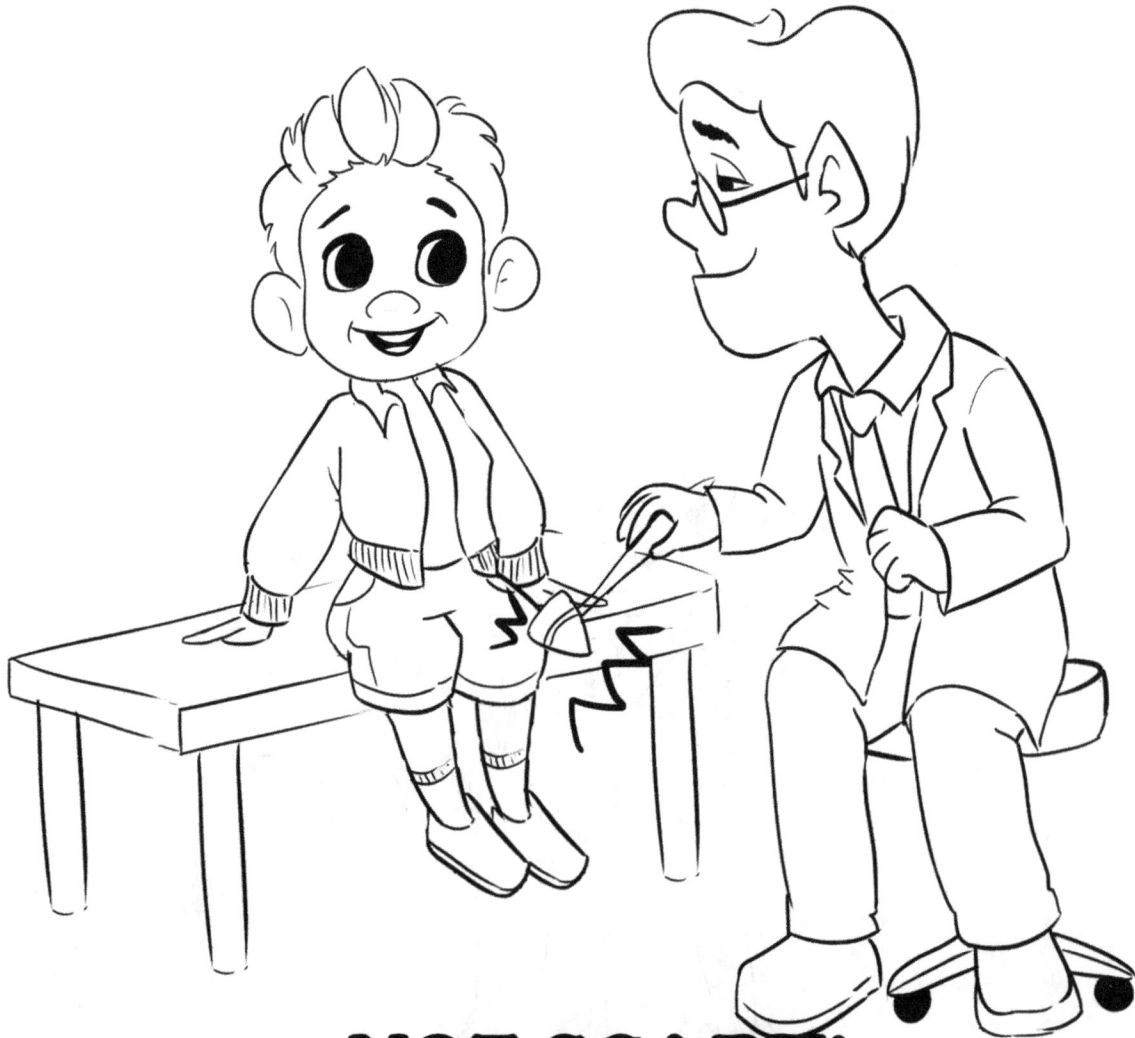

NOT SCARY!

MAGIC STRINGS

(stitches)

Everybody gets cuts sometimes. Some are bigger than others. Often a bandage like this can help it heal. Sometimes the doctor uses Magic Strings to keep the edges together.

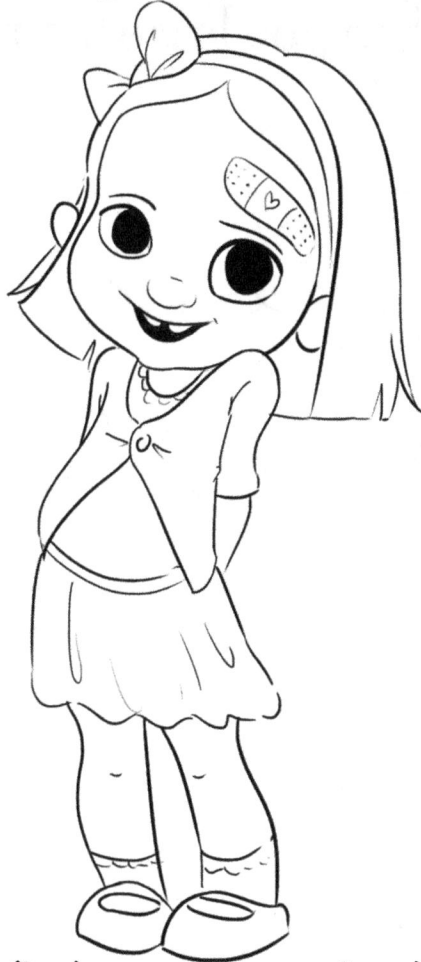

(let's say it together)
NOT SCARY!

CAST

There is even a hard kind of bandage called A CAST. It holds your broken arm or leg still so it can heal. It can be pretty colors, and some people like to have their friends draw on it or write their names! The doctor wraps it around and around, then it gets hard like your play-dough when you leave it out. It doesn't hurt and it's

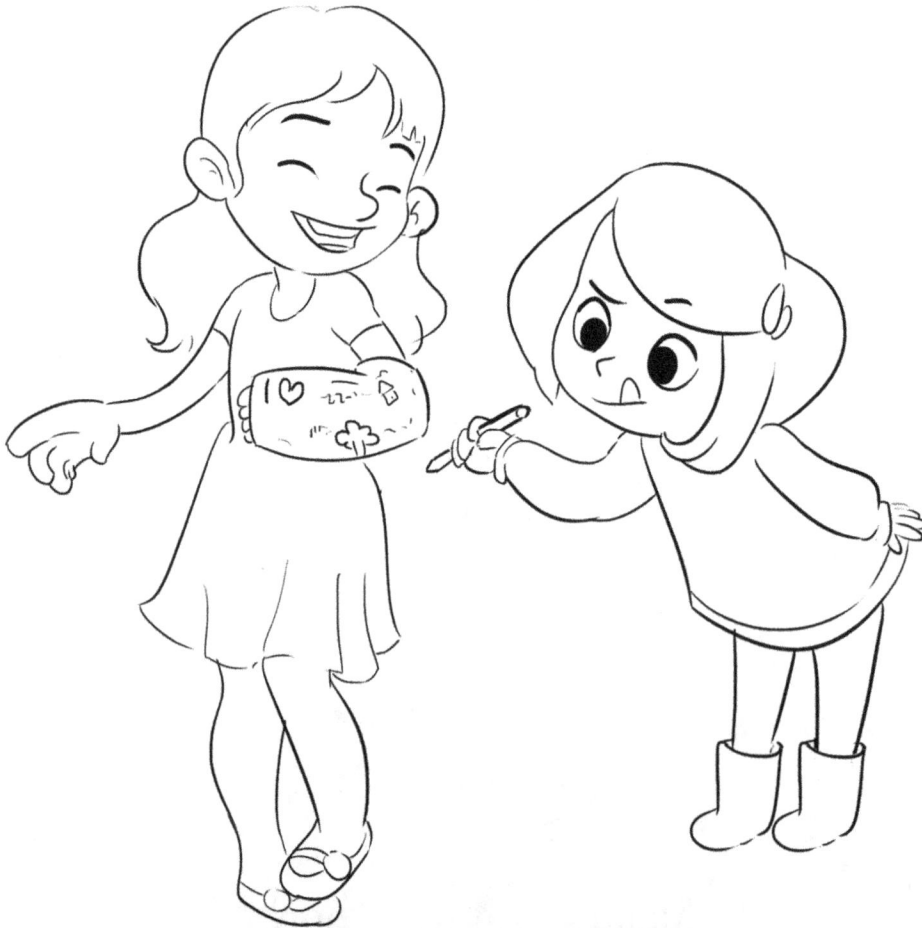

NOT SCARY!

We're at the end of the visit! You were so brave... And you helped others feel strong and safe. Going to the doctor is

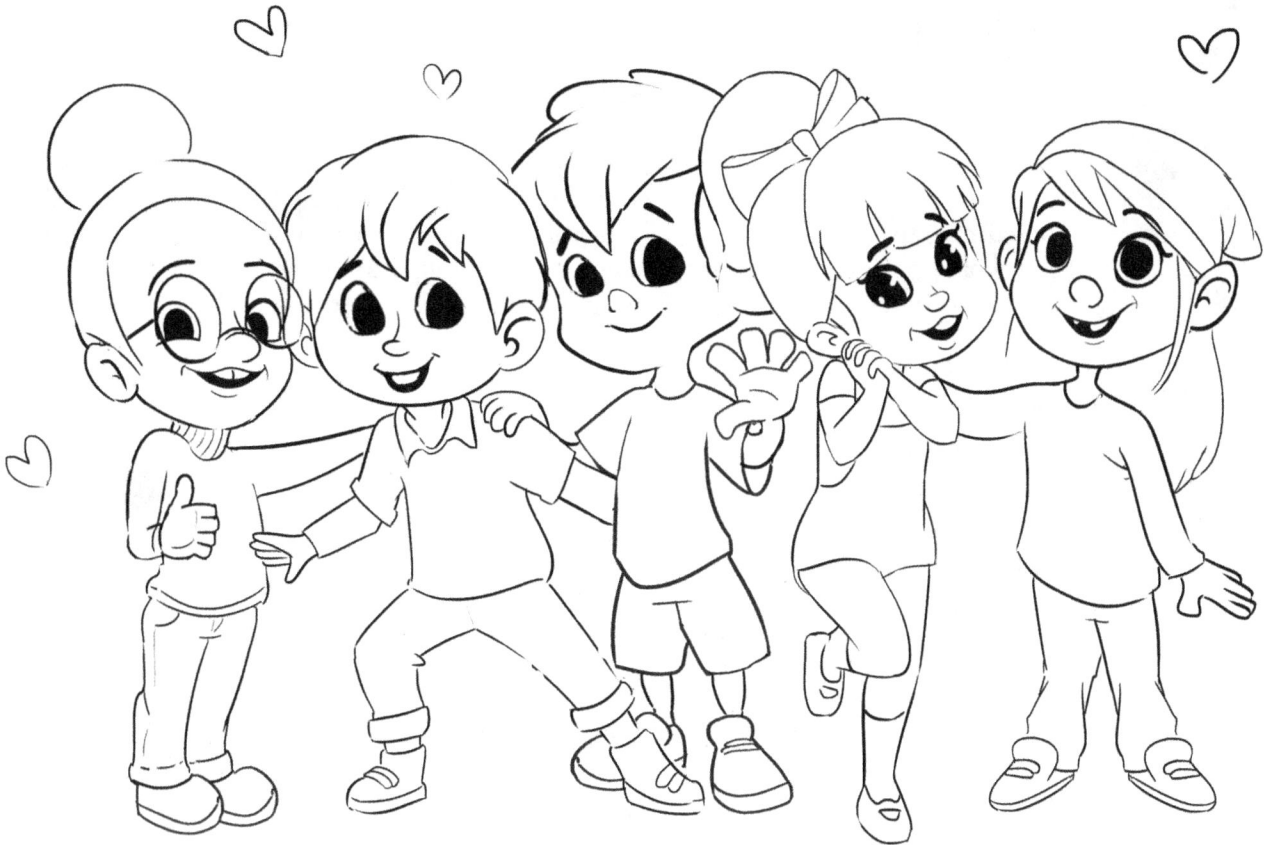

(say it loud and proud)

NOT SCARY!

About the Author

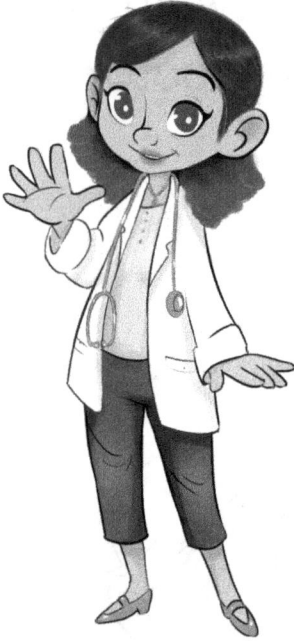

Tana Holmes is the author and creator of beautifully illustrated and creatively constructed books for children of all ages. She is best known for The History Tree Series, where the story-telling tree asks the young reader, "If old trees could talk, what tales could they tell?" The Old Patriarch Tree is set in Holmes' native Wyoming, in Grand Teton National Park. The Dueling Oak relates tales of New Orleans since its founding, and her best-known work, Alamo Tree has earned high praise from Texas historians, teachers, and parents alike. The unique use of easy reader combined with "Reader Guidance" footnotes helps the adult reader enrich the content as the child's development warrants.

Holmes' new series, The NOT Scary Books, uses fantasy and familiar experiences to create tear-free, fear-free adventures out of first-time visits. The unknowns of the doctor, the dentist, daycare, and other dreaded outings have changed from fearful, to fascinating and fun.

Mrs. Holmes has a background in emergency medicine and public administration prior to choosing a career as a health science educator. Entering her 3rd decade of teaching medicine to high school and college students, she divides her time between teaching and authorship. Home is Houston, Texas with her firefighter husband and two rescue dogs. Her adult daughter and son in law are not far away in Austin.

If you enjoyed this book, please consider leaving a review.
For more information about Tana Holmes and her books, please visit
www.historytreeseries.com, or follow her on
Twitter https://twitter.com/history_tree
Facebook https://www.facebook.com/oldtreesrock
Instagram https://www.instagram.com/historytrees/
Goodreads https://www.goodreads.com/author/show/19919054.Tana_S_Holmes
And Amazon https://www.amazon.com/~/e/B083RLLKV6

About the Illustrator

Mahfuja Selim is a freelance illustrator mostly working on Children books for 8 years. She loves creating characters and locations that come from around the world. Her semi-cartoony drawing style sets her apart in the field. Her work has been published throughout the world in children's books, magazines, educational publications, children's games and packaging. She works with modern digital drawing tools at hand combined with all the traditional knowledge. Children love her work.

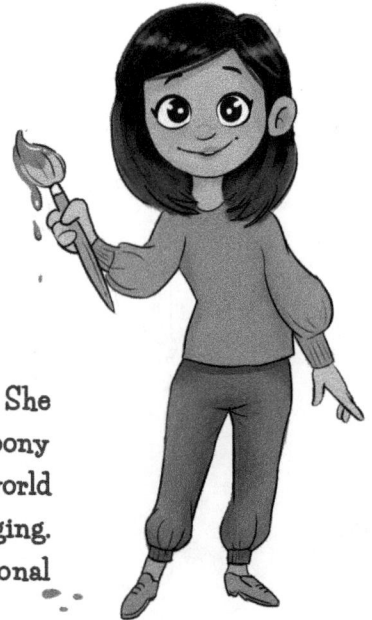

www.ingramcontent.com/pod-product-compliance
Lightning Source LLC
Chambersburg PA
CBHW080349050426

42336CB00053B/3309